I0115711

BARIATRIC EXERCISE

A GENTLE INTRODUCTION TO MOVEMENT PRE- AND POST-SURGERY

MARCOS HERNANDEZ

CONTENTS

FOREWORD

WELCOME. To the start of your new journey. I congratulate you on Day 1 of potential change rather than just waiting on one day in the future to change. The fact that you have chosen to read this e-book doesn't necessarily mean that you will follow through with the goal you may have set for yourself, but what it does indicate is that you have enough interest in investigating the possibilities of what could be a new change for you.

Here are a few questions that I would like for you to ponder while construing this book: your purpose, your commitment, and your maintenance of results. While this book is meant to encourage you, it will not provide you the responses to the aforementioned points. Rather this book should be used as a framework for your health and wellness blueprint. This document has been written with the consideration that you may not possess any technical knowledge in diet, metabolism, and motion. The words have been written to inform you of certain processes and management of your self in such a way you will want to know more and do more for you.

I met and became a student of Marcos Antonio Hernandez in 2017–
only after making a deal with my then fifteen-year-old son–that I
would seek a personal trainer and attempt to lose the weight before
heading off to having Sleeve Gastrectomy surgery performed in
Mexico. Our first meeting was contentious; I believed Marcos and me
to be a mismatched pair. He was young, and I was mature. He was fit,
and I was urban-voluptuous (thick). He was intellect, and I sassy.
However, in hindsight, I believe that it was just my conscientious
realization that I had indeed selected a personal training partner who
was not going to allow me to fail myself. Marcos and I embarked on a
journey that was marked with early morning training twice a week,
which endure today.

IN THE BEGINNING, THERE WAS PAIN. HE PUSHED, AND I PUSHED BACK.

...with 242 pounds on my 5-foot 5-inch frame and forty-four years
old. I was not a CrossFit-ready spring chicken. No Samantha Briggs
here. I was in poor health. 3X in shirts and size 18 in pants. Pre-
diabetic, hypertensive, vertigo caused by a positional disorder, irreg-
ular bowels, a highly stressed life, poor diet with excessive drinking
and partying. My weight hid insecurities, abuse, rejections, and many
fears. Note to self; it is definitely about what was eating me.

With Marcos's guidance, I gradually became re-acquainted with
balance, posture, and position. Our workouts were meant to focus on
moving and keeping me safe. We squatted, we swung kettlebells, we
bear crawled and, in the beginning, we ended a lot of our sessions
with a simple walk on the street, lined with warehouses. To me, my
trainer became Christmas. There was a gift given to me in each of the
sessions, just like the gift you have received by coming by way of this
manual. It was not a match made in heaven because of anything
Marcos did, but it was more of a silent commitment to not give up on
getting me back to being well. Over the years, Marcos continues to

demonstrate the uncanny ability to understand what regimens would work, and even with me not adhering to a strict eating schedule, and being diagnosed with a frozen shoulder, I have been able to build incredible strength through weight lifting, squatting and HIIT exercises.

Marcos and I trained together up and until my surgery in 2019 and picked back up after my return from Mexico 6 weeks later, and even in a pandemic, I continue to train with him using a customized plan.

Very briefly, I want to mention that weight loss surgery of any kind is not a permanent solution but rather one tool in your toolbox of many other instruments that can be used in your reconstruction to good health. Nor does weight loss represent a quick fix or answer to that which may be in your mind, soul, and wellness regimen. What weight loss surgery offers is the ability to create a new physical reality for your body, but that still does not offer wellness. What we know is wellness comes from an overall sense of your Being's totality.

THE OUTLOOK...

Admittedly I do not confess to be a lover of the gym, but I do have respect for my trainer who has invested so much in training me. Today at 14 months post-op, I am 75 pounds lighter, several dress-sizes smaller, and much healthier than I have been in the last 25 years.

Marcos has skillfully crafted this manual for you; use the information, and trust the process. Take your time while reading, process where you have been and where your current navigation is leading you. Remember that your reflections will be different than everyone else's. No two roads are the same. My words are meant (just like this book) to inspire you to see your change through. Wherever you should end up on your journey, always stay authentic.

Congratulations and cheers!

Alarice Vidale de Palacios

Director, Applied Bariatric Counseling

May 2020

WELCOME

OVERVIEW

SO YOU'VE DECIDED bariatric surgery is right for you but don't know what to do to prepare. Or perhaps you've already undergone the procedure and want to learn how to move as your body changes.

You want to put yourself in the best possible position for success. At the end of the tunnel is a version of you with less baggage, one who will be able to move around the world with new-found ease.

The strategy for learning to move your body both before AND after your surgery is the same. The principles don't change. It's a slow, measured response to a new challenge: how to get active.

Moving can seem daunting. But anything outside of your comfort zone seems that way until you trust a guide to show you the path.

You might not know where to begin.. But that's OK! Learning to manipulate your body in space is a challenge worth undertaking.

You've done the research, checked out books (like this one!), tried the diets and exercise plans. I'm here to help you cut through the noise.

Luke had Yoda before he became a Jedi. I'm not small, nor green, but I can still help show the way.

Let this book be your guide on the path.

How do you get started? Well, I've got news for you: you started the moment you began reading this book. In the following pages, I'll lay out an easy to digest guide to human movement that is both accessible and comprehensive.

Have you ever heard the saying about how to eat an elephant? One bite at a time.

Learning to move is much the same way. One step at a time, over a long time, produces results that aren't a flash in the pan, they're the kind that sticks around for the long haul. This is because this book doesn't just lay out a quick exercise strategy, it's a guide to teach you how your body is designed to move in space.

I'm passionate about movement and hope that one day you can be too.

YOU CAN DO THIS

YOU MIGHT WANT to wait until the weight is already gone to get started on your movement journey. But what if I told you there is still a LOT you can learn before then?

If you take the time to learn early on, you can make more significant progress once there's less of you to move. The patterns in this book are an introduction, made for people just like you, who have decided bariatric surgery is right for them.

What I want you to understand is this: you can learn how to move regardless of your physical size. Don't let the images of people you see as "typical" exercisers affect your opinion of your abilities. Humans are designed with the same basic structure, so age and physical size don't change whether you can perform the moves in this book.

Take a step back. You picked up a book about training! That's a HUGE win. Let that sink in. Appreciate it. Would previous versions of yourself do something like this?

I have a request: read this book in its entirety. At least look at the pictures and see the logic behind how you will learn to move. Over time, these same moves will become more relaxed and will lead to more complex variations.

By all means, take breaks between chapters or sections. Try out the movements that speak to you. But try, really try, to get through all the material. I've made it short and sweet on purpose because I care about your success and want you to be exposed to these concepts.

It's possible to learn how to move in YOUR body, regardless of physical size. My hope for you is that you learn to enjoy it!

Then, armed with your newfound appreciation for movement, moving with less weight won't be a chore... it will be exciting!

WRITE YOUR OWN STORY

STILL NOT SURE if this is for you?

I have a feeling we both want this book to work.

But you'll have to let go of any preconceived notions you have about exercising and look at this from the perspective of learning how to *move.*

If you've tried an exercise routine before, please don't let that color you're mindset going into reading this book. Give it a shot with an open mind!

The hardest part will be the first time you try out the first suggested movements. Inertia is tough to get over, but I believe you can do it.

Find the time to give it a go. What do you have to lose?

I'll also provide some advice on building the habit at the end of the book. Over time, my hope is to give you a different outlook on movement, showing you that it doesn't have to be intimidating.

Your future is right around the corner. Ready to lay the groundwork?

INTRO TO THE BODY

BREATHING

THERE'S a good chance your movement options are limited, regardless of whether you've already gotten the surgery or it's upcoming.

But the fact that you're reading this book is a good sign you're serious about getting started. It can be daunting, but I am going to make the transition to working on movement as easy as possible.

You can get started right where you are.

The first step to learning how to move your body begins with breathing.

THE BREATH

Why should you care about breathing? Well, if your surgery hasn't been performed yet, a genuine concern for anesthesiologists is how to properly ventilate obese surgery patients due to the reduced lung volume. [1]

If your surgery has already been performed, an improvement in breathing mechanics will help once exercise becomes more strenuous.

The goal in both scenarios is to increase the amount of air in the lungs. More air = more oxygen getting to your body.

A study found that subjects who suffered from chronic obstructive pulmonary disease (COPD) who performed diaphragmatic breathing showed an increase in lung volume. [2]

From the U.S. National Library of Medicine: "The diaphragm, located below the lungs, is the major muscle of respiration. It is a large, dome-shaped muscle that contracts rhythmically and continually, and most of the time, involuntarily. Upon inhalation, the diaphragm contracts and flattens and the chest cavity enlarges. This contraction creates a vacuum, which pulls air into the lungs. Upon exhalation, the diaphragm relaxes and returns to its domelike shape, and air is forced out of the lungs." [3]

Put simply, the goal is to get the diaphragm moving while you breathe.

How? By *breathing through your nose.*

NASAL BREATHING

In a study comparing diaphragm movement during both mouth-breathing and nasal-breathing, it was found that the diaphragm moved much less during mouth-breathing. [4]

I'm imagining that you're trying to breathe through your nose now. Hopefully, it isn't too uncomfortable!

Let me provide some structure so you can learn to get comfortable breathing through your nose. This technique is called "box breathing."

First, think about breathing in four parts:

1. Inhale
2. Inhale hold
3. Exhale
4. Exhale hold

What I want you to do is make each of these four parts equal, all while breathing through your nose. It's OK if you need to open your mouth... we're learning after all!

Start with one second at each part, performing it for five breaths. Then, rest and breathe in a way comfortable for you.

When you're ready to try again, try performing five breaths, taking two seconds at each part. The goal is to work up to performing five breaths with five seconds spent at each. That exhale hold gets spicy, so don't be surprised if you struggle!

The goal would be to do this protocol at least once a day, but it could be done more frequently if you have the time and desire. Some useful places to insert this breathing practice into your day might be right after you wake up, during a quick break before you get out of the car, or before bed.

There's lots of quality work you can do without getting up from where you are. Bet you didn't think the movement of your diaphragm would count as learning to move!

Taking the time to work on breathing will set you up for success down the line, both for bariatric surgery and for the active lifestyle beyond.

Now you've got a starting point to launch from and tangible evidence that you can do this!

BODY SCAN

YOU'VE MASTERED (or attempted) the breathing method described in the previous chapter. You're feeling good, feeling inspired, and ready to move some muscles.

So let's get moving! *One body part at a time.*

The goal of this section is to discover if you have any pain. If any of these suggestions cause you to experience pain, please contact a physical therapist. I work closely with the team at Cohen Health and Performance (CHP) and know they would be happy to help. They're based in the D.C./Maryland area, but they offer remote services for those further away.

It's time to meet the rest of your body.

The first part of your body we will review in this section is closely related to the nasal breathing patterns we already went over: the tongue.

THE TONGUE

What does the tongue have to do with breathing, you ask? Why let me tell you!

A study found that children who breathed through their mouths had less tongue strength than their nasal breathing counterparts. [5] The study concludes, "The breathing pattern impacts tongue pressure development." We can work backward, hoping to affect some change in breathing patterns by strengthening the tongue.

If that's not enough reason for you, strengthening the tongue can also help you sleep better. A common cause of obstructive sleep apnea is the collapse of the upper airway brought about by a reduction in tongue-muscle activity. One study found that increasing tongue strength while a person is awake affects their ability to keep the airway open while asleep. [6]

I want you to try and move your tongue in two ways. Try both out, ten times each:

1. Press the entire tongue against the roof of your mouth. Imagine you're sucking on a piece of hard candy.
2. Press the tip of your tongue into the highest part of the roof of your mouth. Imagine your trying to touch the tip of your nose from the inside.

You can also do these exercises as holds, shooting for five seconds of pressing as hard as you can.

MEETING YOUR BODY

Now that we've gotten that out of the way, it's time to move your joints. We'll start from the top, focusing on the upper body first:

Neck. These movements begin with the eyes, followed by the head:

- Look to the left and turn to the left, look to the right and turn to the right
- Look up, then lift your chin, look down, then tuck your chin (try and see the collar of your shirt).
- In a neutral position, push your chin forward as far as you can
- In a neutral position, pull your chin back. It helps to think about touching the wall behind you with the back of your head.

Shoulders:

- Reach forward, toward the wall across from you, as far as you can
- Lift your arms up and reach to the ceiling
- Lift your arms to the sides and reach to the walls on your left and right

Elbows:

- Make your arms as straight as possible, attempting to lock the elbow
- Bend both arms, like you're doing a curl, with the palms up
- Bend both arms with the palms down

Wrists. Make a fist with both hands then:

- Crank your wrists down, like starting a motorcycle.
- Turn your wrists back, with your first knuckles pointing to the ceiling
- In a neutral position, turn your fist both left and right
- To challenge yourself, try hitting these positions in continuous circles

Once you've tried out those positions, it's time to move to the lower body. We're going to start at the bottom and work our way up for these joint movements:

Ankles. Try these one side at a time:

- Point your toes and reach forward as far as you can
- Lift your toes up and pull them towards your knees
- In a neutral position, turn your foot left and right
- To challenge yourself, try hitting these positions in continuous circles

Knees. These moves will be performed from a seated position:

- Straighten your leg as much as possible, attempting to lock the knee
- Sitting on the edge of the chair, bend your knee as much as possible

Hips. You'll need to lay down for this:

- Lift one leg at a time, bending at the hip. You don't need to keep your leg straight.

It's common for individuals with excess weight to compensate for muscle weaknesses and instability by altering joint loading patterns. [7] These repetitive patterns of joint misalignment, when combined with the elevated inflammation associated with obesity, can lead to pain in the joints. [8,9]

By choosing to undergo bariatric surgery, you're addressing both the cause of altered joint loading patterns and the underlying cause of inflammation. But the movement piece can't be overlooked! One study found that COPD patients with elevated levels of inflammation benefited from physical activity. [10]

So, taking each joint through its range of motion addresses address both issues that could lead to pain: loading patterns and elevated inflammation.

THE PLAN

It does take a while to work through all the movements listed above. Who knew there were so many ways your body could move! An effective way I've found to get people to get through it all is to set a five-minute timer and work through as many movements as possible. Try this out a couple of times a day and see how far you get.

Some of these positions might be challenging, so take your time. There might be some limitations you were unaware of. Again, if you feel pain in any area, please consult a physical therapist.

This is an actionable introduction to the ways your joints can move, one that lays the groundwork for the movements in upcoming sections. With this increased knowledge, see if you can spot some parts in your day when you're stuck in a particular position. Maybe your neck is stiff after staring at a screen all day, or your knee is tight from being propped up... now you know what each of these joints is capable of and how to get them moving!

EXERCISE FAMILY 1 - BELOW THE HIPS

SINGLE LEG BALANCE

WHETHER YOU'RE PREPARING for bariatric surgery or have recently undergone the procedure, there's a good chance you have limited mobility. Just getting up and into the other room may pose its own challenge. For those recovering, you may find that just standing up is enough some days.

The goal is to regain as much mobility as possible, one step at a time. More exercise options will become available to you as you learn to move without restriction. It just takes time and practice.

Since the distance from a couch or chair might be a concern, we're going to start close to your home base. I want you to feel safe as you undertake the process of learning how to move.

STANDING TALL

The first thing we are going to work on is balance. Stand up with your feet straight ahead and feel your body from the ground up. Find the stability in your feet, find the muscles around your knees and hips working to keep you upright.

Try and keep your shoulders over your hips, your hips over your ankles.

Then, once you're ready, we're going to progress to balancing on one foot. Start by putting one foot slightly in front of the other, lining up your heel with your toes. Then shift your weight to your back foot.

Once you're comfortable with the majority of your weight on your back foot, try and lift your front foot.

Try and hold this for ten seconds on both sides to start. The goal is to work up to thirty seconds on both sides.

If you need to rest between attempts, do so.

THE IMPORTANCE OF BALANCE

Several studies draw a link between obesity and a lack of balance. The first studied sixty young adults and found the feet of obese individuals pointed out more than those with a lower BMI. [11] Greater angles in the feet have been shown to affect balance and the risk of falling, even in populations without underlying health issues. [12]

A second study that measured balance among older women (approximately seventy years old) also found that obesity had an effect on their ability to balance. [13] This study is especially relevant for older bariatric surgery patients

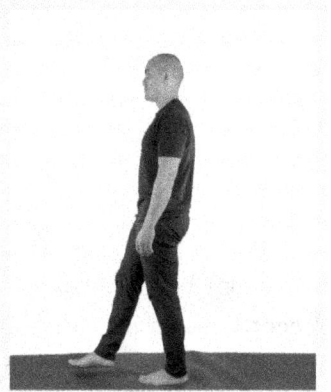

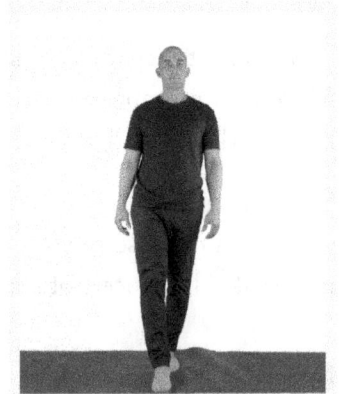

because the potential damage from a fall is more significant for older individuals.

Since spending time in an obese body has been linked with balance limitations, it's crucial to work on this skill. This holds true even if you've already undergone bariatric surgery and have begun your journey towards a smaller version of yourself.

The couch or chair behind you might still be calling your name while you practice. If you find yourself discouraged, take a break, and try again later! Learning to move well is a lengthy process; it's better to keep your eyes on the horizon instead of forcing movement all at once.

Working on this skill doesn't require much of your time. You could start with performing this movement during commercials, or between shows. The trick is to find enough times to practice throughout the day, so you're getting up and moving as much as possible, useful for both pre- and post-surgery.

Don't be surprised when the thirty-second recommendation above turns into a minute at a time on each leg!

Now that you know it's possible to move without going into a separate space, how can you add this move into your daily life?

STAND UP, SIT DOWN

YOU MAY FEEL TIED to the couch if your weight makes it difficult to move. Or, if you're recovering from surgery, you have to take it easy while your limited food intake saps your energy.

The future holds a version of yourself able to move around with ease, taking long walks if you choose.

The first step is getting up from your chair or bed.

I know what you're thinking: why would getting up come *after* the section on balance. That doesn't make any sense! Don't you have to stand up before working on balance in the first place?

Well, the goal of this exercise is to get up and get back down *multiple times*. When you went through the balance section, you only had to get up a single time. Once you were standing, all you had to do was... well, stand there!

STAND UP, SIT DOWN

There are four ways we are going to work standing up and sitting back down.

Version 1 - Reaching, with a chair:

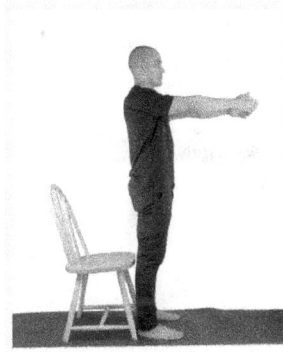

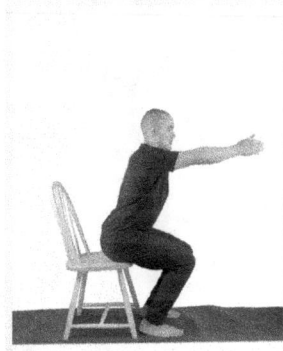

Try and get back to standing five times.

Reach as far as you can when you're performing this version. Imagine you're trying to grab something from the furthest corner of a shelf. It's an active position, not just arms ahead!

As you lower yourself to the chair, try and limit the amount of weight you put onto the chair. Think of it as a depth marker. Once you find the chair, you stand right back up, collect your balance, and try again.

Version 2 - Hands in, with a chair:

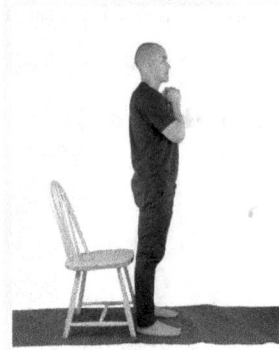

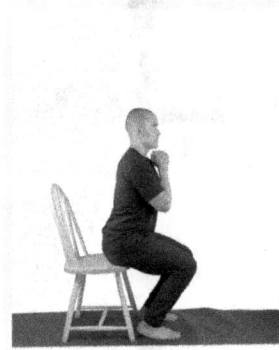

Try and get back to standing five times.

While performing this version, keep your hands together at the base of your neck. Your fingers can be interlocked, you could bring two fists together, or have your palms meet in a praying position.

Try to keep your elbows as close together as possible while you do this.

Version 3 - Reaching, without chair:

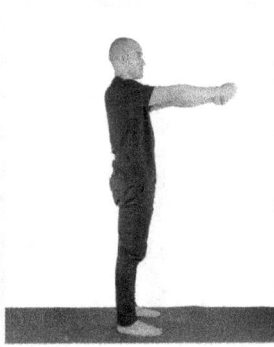

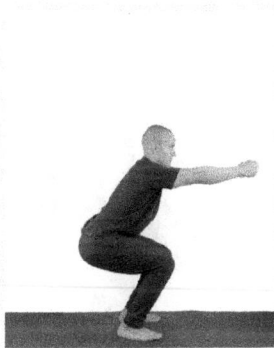

Try and get back to standing five times.

In this version, we're taking away the support. The goal is to get back to the exact same level as the chair, all while actively reaching away.

Version 4 - Hands in, without chair:

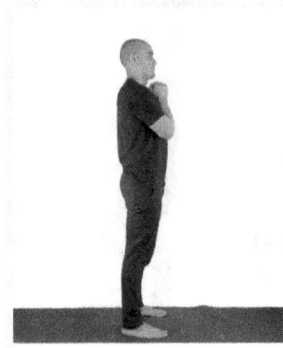

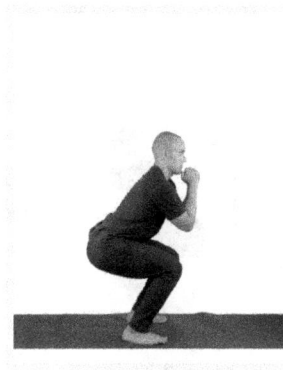

Try and get back to standing five times.

Again, hands together at the base of your neck. This is the most challenging version, so give yourself a break if you find it too challenging and need to go back to a different version.

There's a chance your body will want to stop you before you reach the height of the chair when doing all four of these variations. If this happens, take a couple deep breaths through your nose and try again. As you get to the height where you begin to slow down, slowly exhale. The hope is that your body will relax enough to allow you to get down to the correct height.

A link has been made between a reduction in leg strength and obesity. [14] By standing up and sitting back down, you are building the strength in your legs needed as you regain mobility and begin to move around more frequently.

GETTING INTO THE ROUTINE

There might be some pain at first, particularly in your ankles, knees, and hips. If it's mild, take some time before trying again. Don't push through pain! Just make a promise to yourself that you'll come back later, or tomorrow, and try again.

If the pain is intense and/or persists, get in contact with a physical therapist.

It's going to take some time to get through these four versions of standing up and sitting back down. Make a promise to yourself that you'll come back and keep trying, every day or a few times a week. If you can work up to standing up ten times, multiple times per day, you're doing great!

Plus, by taking the time to get better at this pattern, you're proving you can keep a promise to yourself regarding movement. It's all about learning to layer quality movement consistently into your daily life.

Armed with these four variations and the knowledge that lasting fitness isn't built in a day, you're well on your way to turning a weakness into a strength!

PAUSED MARCHING

YOU'VE HEARD of crawl before you can walk, right? Well, I'd like to add a step before walking. A crawling and a half if you will.

The goal is to add a little more movement into the routine, another step after balancing and standing up. Enter: marching.

When carrying excess weight or recovering from surgery, walking isn't as straightforward as going outside and getting after it.

Marching is useful because you get to stay close to your couch or chair, the supports you'll need when it's time to rest.

If you've been able to incorporate the other two movements into your routine, you're already familiar with the challenge of getting started. It's easy to stay still and wait until the weight is gone. But there are steps you can take (literally!) to set you up for success in the future.

MARCHING

Try for ten marches, five per leg, rest, then repeat three times.

Raise your knees as high as you can. A way to challenge yourself would be to add in a pause when your knee is at its highest point. It's ok if your knee doesn't get anywhere close to what you see in the photo—as you get better, you'll find that you can raise your knees higher and higher.

Keeping your arms up isn't required, but it does help build some strength in your shoulders and arms. Do whatever you need to keep your balance. We'll revisit the upper body in later sections.

A study performed in 2016 found that obese individuals who participated in a walking routine had a reduction in body weight and waist circumference while increasing their muscular strength. [15] Marching in place is a safe first step to being able to walk and will have similar benefits.

ADDING IT TO THE MIX

As with the other exercises you'll find in this book, it's important not to do too much on your first attempt. It's better to sit back down and rest while you feel like you still have more in the tank. You can always try again later!

One thing to keep in mind as you begin to move your body is that there often might be a delay in the onset of effects. I'm not implying you believe you'll get the entire benefits of

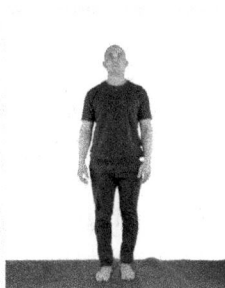

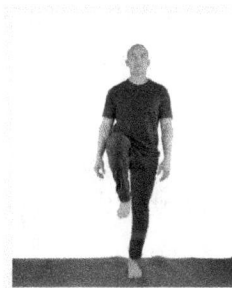

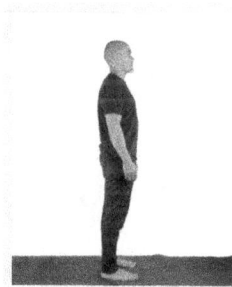

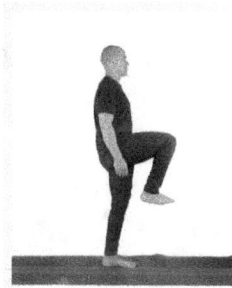

walking on the first day; instead, this warning is more about things like muscle soreness and cramps. These sometimes take a full day to show up, so it's better to rest at the end of your session and see how your body is affected.

Focus on being ready to try again tomorrow. Then the next day. And the day after that.

One trick that helps enforce the habit is to cross off the days on a calendar that you move. If you get a few days in a row, there's an incentive to move and keep the streak alive. Keeping the streak alive is a powerful motivation tool when you don't feel like exercising!

With marching, you can work on walking without leaving the comfort of the supports you have in your home. Try it out!

STANDING KNEE BENDS

YOU WANT TO EXERCISE, move around, get active, but knee pain after standing up makes it so you have to rest sooner than you'd like. This is a common issue for patients both before and after bariatric surgery.

Being able to stand longer without knee pain would allow you to spend more time practicing the exercises in this book and improve your mobility. This could make even something like a simple grocery store more bearable.

A study found that obese individuals walk slower than non-obese participants, and another found that knee pain is more common among people who walk at a slower pace. [16,17]

So knee pain can be traced back to a slower walking speed! And a slower walking speed means more time is spent on your feet whenever you do need to be mobile.

On the flip side, a study found that obese individuals with knee pain relied on locking their knees while standing, which could be the cause of discomfort. [18]

Time on your feet doesn't have to be the enemy. By taking the time to work on bending the knee with purpose and attention, we can strengthen the muscles responsible for the action. This leads to more control, and more control allows your knee to have more movement options whenever life does call for you to be standing for any length of time.

STANDING KNEE BENDS

The goal of this movement is to practice bending the knee in a controlled manner. See if you can pause at the top of the rep, holding it for a quick second before letting your foot lower under control.

Shoot for five reps per leg, rest, and repeat.

Like with the paused marching, you'll be able to lift your leg higher as you get more practice with this move.

ABOUT THE PRACTICE

You might notice some cramping in the back of the leg. This is ok and completely normal. If your leg does cramp up, sit down and try again tomorrow. These are just the muscles in the back of the leg getting used to moving again. The development of these muscles will help you control the bending of your knee over time.

Once cramping has begun, there isn't any more you can do that day, since the same issue will come up again and again. Several

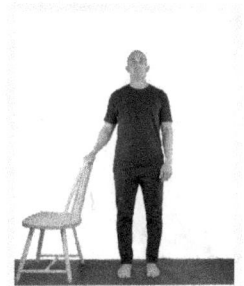

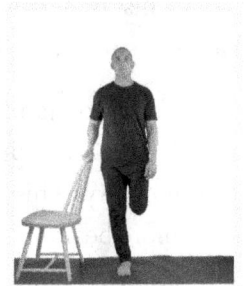

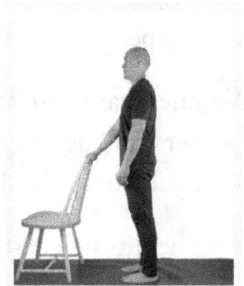

factors contribute to cramping, but the best way to combat and alleviate cramping is to drink water. Electrolyte water, if possible.

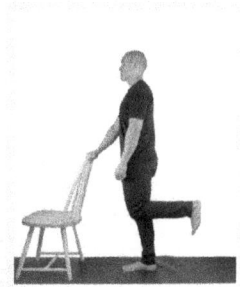

On the topic of drinking water, try and keep a water bottle within arms reach throughout the day. Don't get hung up on the specific amount of water you drink just consume as much as you comfortably can. One client discovered that what he had assumed was hunger before turned out to be thirst. By adding in a steady amount of water each day and drinking water before meals, he was able to reduce the amount of food he ate at each meal.

Put simply, drinking water can have a direct effect on your ability to work on your movement each day. Try stacking both habits and see how many days in a row you can practice this move!

BENDING AT THE HIP

HAVE you ever suffered from lower back pain?

You aren't alone. A study of over nine hundred men published in 2016 found that high intensity lower back pain was associated with increased levels of obesity. [19]

The onset of lower back pain is a common issue among obese individuals when starting a movement practice. This could be because of the stiffness of the spine. A study published in the *Journal of Neurosurgery* found that lumbar spinal segments from obese donors seem to behave differently upon the testing of biomechanics measurements. [20]

It must be noted that lower back pain is a complex issue, and several psychosocial factors have been reported as risk factors. These include stress, anxiety, and job dissatisfaction. [21]

But there's hope! By learning how to properly bend at the hip, you'll provide your body with increased movement options in the affected area. More movement options mean less stiffness!

Below are the steps you can take to learn to bend at the hip that will minimize the forces on your lower back. If this family of moves **does** cause pain, contact a physical therapist.

BENDING AT THE HIP

This is the first movement where you will have to orient your body in space horizontally. In the previous drills, the forces were vertical, meaning we could use the ground to know the direction we had to push away from.

We're going to use the wall, or a heavy piece of furniture, in the first two variations, so your body has an outside surface to reference.

Version 1 - Reaching, finding the wall

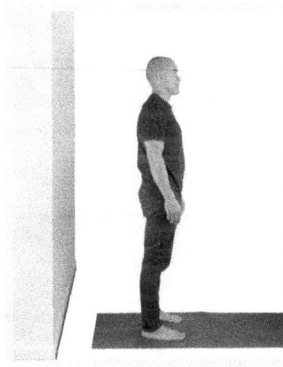

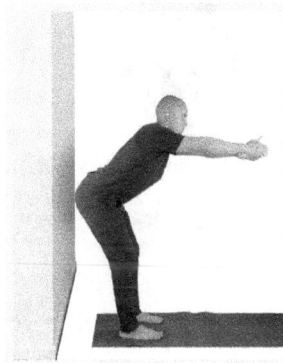

Start with your heels just a few inches from the wall, shift your weight back in your heels, and find the wall behind you. Try not to have your knees locked. If this is easy, step forward a bit and try again.

Try to lightly touch the wall five times.

The reaching we practiced in the "Stand Up, Sit Down" section is back for this drill. Not only are you reaching forward with your hands, think about reaching back with your backside until you find the wall. You should feel a slight stretch in the back of your legs, but don't worry if not, everyone's body responds differently.

Version 2 - Hands in, finding the wall

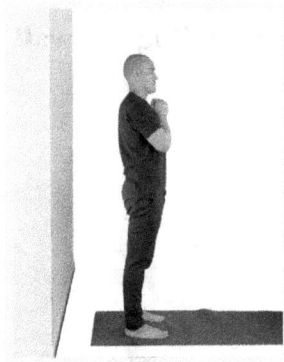

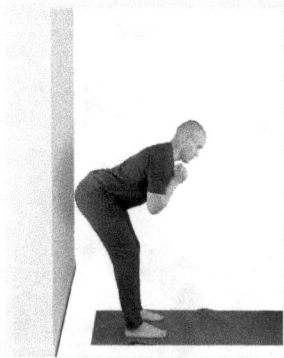

This one is a bit more challenging because you don't have the counterweight provided by your arms. The same thing as before, Start with your heels just a few inches from the wall, shift your weight back in your heels, and find the wall behind you without locking your knees. If this is easy, step forward a bit and try again.

Try to lightly touch the wall five times.

Version 3 - Reaching, in space

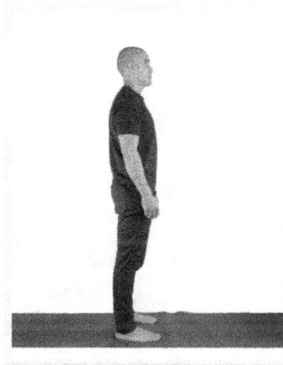

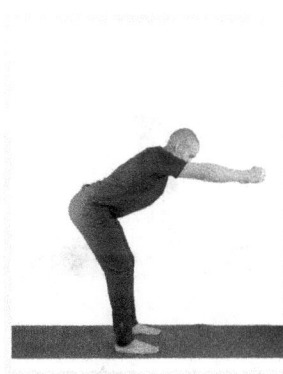

Time to kick things up a notch and take away the wall. Actively reach forward with your hands while you reach behind you with your backside. You don't have to go far on this one! Remember how we started with this pattern in the first place, just a few inches off the wall. Shift your weight onto your heels and try a small movement first, return to standing, then try and get a bit farther back as you become more comfortable.

Try to reach behind you five times.

Version 4 - Hands in, in space

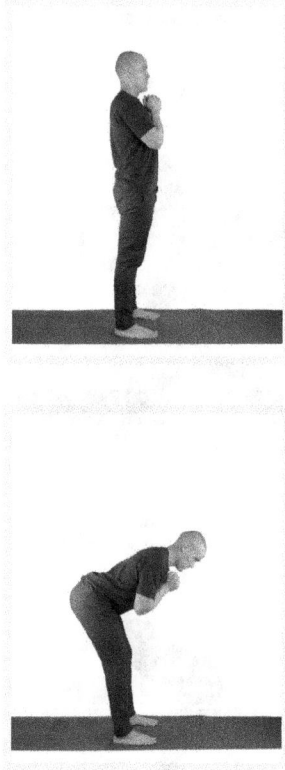

This is the hardest version. Feel free to give it a go once you've worked your way through the progression!

ABOUT BENDING AT THE HIP

This movement requires more focus than the previous ones. The others have a certain amount of "just get it done" while there's more to bending at the hip than just touching the wall with your butt. Take the time to pay attention to what you're doing, feeling your weight shift as you find the wall. Keep in mind, we aren't resting on the wall, just using it as a marker for when we need to change direction.

Learning about the ways your body can move combined with an increase in awareness of what's happening while you do so will provide your body with more movement options. More movement options can decrease stiffness in affected areas and help with chronic pain.

With these tools in your toolkit, it's time to move onto the other half of your body!

EXERCISE FAMILY 2 - ABOVE THE HIPS

SHOULDERS

A LOT of time has been spent on the lower half of the body up to this point. Where's the love for the upper body?

Part of the reason I've waited this long to discuss the upper body is because of the number of preconceived notions associated with upper body exercises.

Quick history lesson: a documentary came out in 1977 called "Pumping Iron." In it, a young bodybuilder named Arnold Schwarzenegger shared his journey to winning a bodybuilding competition. You might've heard of him.

Well, this movie transformed the gym-going population into focusing on the *muscles* instead of the *movement*. This is where the focus on chest, arm, and back muscles entered the mainstream and colored the ideas of upper body exercises for generations.

Up to this point, we haven't seen a single weight. This is deliberate! These upper body movements also require no external load, but that doesn't mean they aren't effective.

My goal with the previous sections was to show you that the intention of the movement is more important than feeling any particular muscle. It's about *quality*. How'd I do?

Hopefully, well enough that you'll be able to try these exercises out without looking for any particular muscle group. Like before, it's all about the *movement*. Specifically, in the shoulders.

THE FOUR WAYS YOUR SHOULDER CAN MOVE

These movements can all be performed both seated, kneeling, or standing. The goal is to do them standing, with your shoulders over your hips over your ankles.

Lifting your arms part 1 - ahead

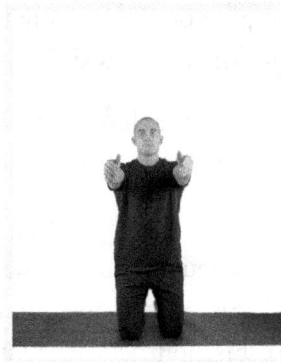

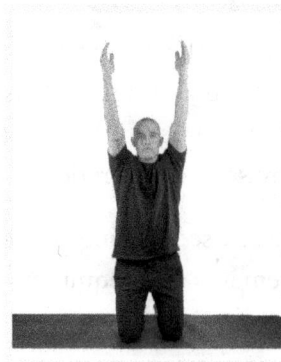

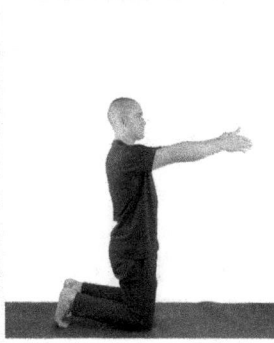

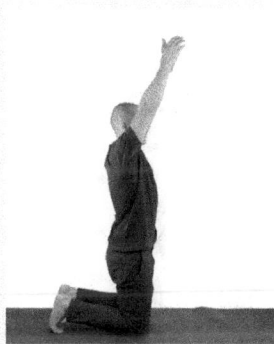

Keep your arms at the same height as you do this. Pause for five seconds with your arms in their highest position and repeat five times.

Lifting your arms part 2 - to the side

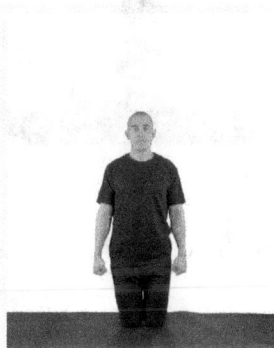

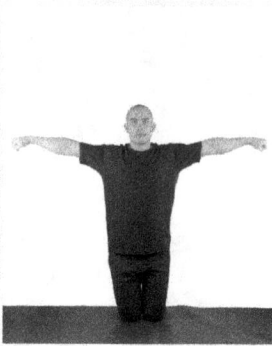

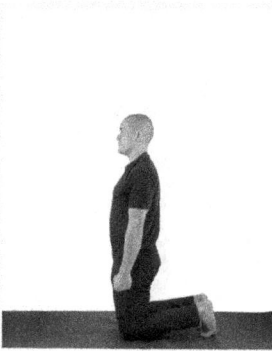

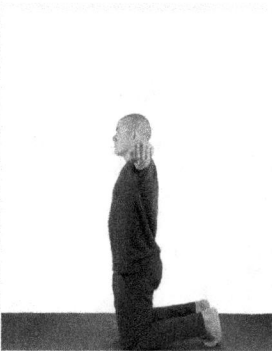

Pause for five seconds with your arms in their highest position and repeat five times.

Squeezing your shoulder blades

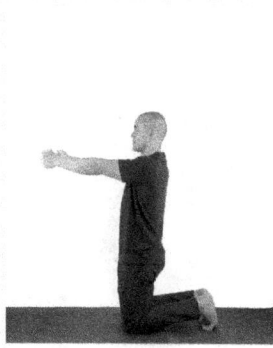

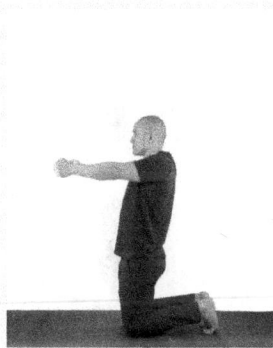

To set up, raise your arms and put the tips of your finger on the wall. Then try and pull your fingers as far away as possible from the wall using your shoulders. If it helps, think about squeezing a pencil between your shoulder blades.

Pause for five seconds with your fingers as far as possible from the wall and repeat five times.

Reaching

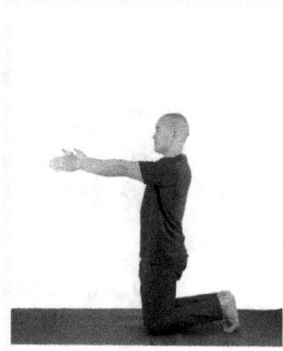

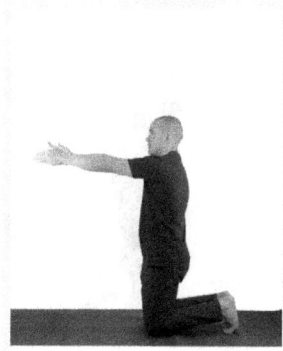

The initial setup for this variation is the same as squeezing your shoulder blades: raise your arms and put the tips of your finger on the wall. This time, take a micro-step back. Try and touch the wall again. Continue this process until your fingers reach an inch or so away from the wall WITHOUT touching the wall.

Pause for five seconds with your arms reaching as far as they can and repeat five times.

This variation is the most dependent on your effort. The change in position will be small, but you have to give it your full attention! Imagine you're reaching for a spice in the furthest corner of your cabinet.

That being said, all four of these variations require you to push yourself. None of them are too challenging if you just get through them. See if you can hold longer, lift higher, or squeeze tighter to get the most benefit from your practice of these.

END RANGES OF MOTION

Are you wondering about the focus on holding the end of the range of motion in the shoulders?

One, it allows us to increase strength without weights. [22]

Two, a study published in 2010 found that out of thirty measured joint ranges of motion, obesity affected one shoulder measure the most. [23]

By taking the time to work on how well your shoulder moves, we are addressing a potential movement limitation that might be present even after bariatric surgery.

The focus on the end range of movement—the hold position in each exercise—is why those positions require so much attention. But the emphasis will pay off once more complex activities become possible in the future.

The fact that we can do so much quality work without weights means there's no barrier to entry. Once your mind is made up, it's time to practice! And since these particular four moves can be performed both seated and standing, they're easier to incorporate into a daily routine.

CORE - FRONTSIDE

IF YOU'RE anything like my clients, you're enjoying a good laugh after reading the title of this section. Go ahead, get it out.

The excess weight around your midsection might be the reason you're getting surgery in the first place!

If you've already undergone the procedure, you might be hesitant to focus on the area that's already tender whenever you eat.

But working on the core is essential, and must be done, so bear with me for a second. I've gotten you this far, haven't I?

Think back to the section about bending at the hip... remember the part about lower back pain? Well, the role of the abdominal muscles is to stabilize the lower back by increasing the amount of pressure inside the system. [24]

So this movement type is worth learning! You should *want* to work on your core. For your back.

Most people immediately think of sit-ups. But these aren't exactly possible with size restrictions or pain limitations around the midsection. So what do we do?

DEAD BUGS

Make sure you keep your head on the floor throughout the movement and shoot to open up each alternating pair three times.

Try and hold your arm and an opposite leg for a quick pause at the end range. It doesn't have to be a long hold, think a second or two, just enough to show control at the position.

Laying on your back with your knees and elbows in the air is the default position. This is where you stay, gather yourself, then try again.

This one plays games with your coordination! Make sure the limbs that aren't moving stay still the entire time. For example, if we are trying to extend our right leg and left arm, our left knee and right elbow should be pointing up to the ceiling.

The benefits of this exercise are two-fold: core stability and coordination. A real bang for your buck exercise!

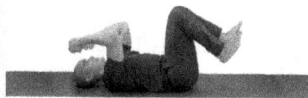

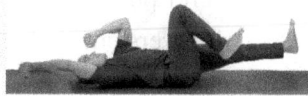

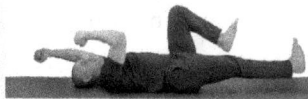

IMPLEMENTATION

Adding these into the mix does add a new component: getting onto the ground. Pick a carpeted area with plenty of space and some sturdy furniture nearby you can use when it's time to get back to standing.

It's ok if they feel awkward. These are challenging for everyone, and it takes time to get used to moving alternating limbs.

For those who have undergone bariatric surgery: take your time and check in with your body while doing these. There are lots of other exercises we can do if there is any "pulling" in your midsection what-soever. Shoot me an email, and I'd love to help you find a solution!

If you get to the point that you feel like you need to challenge yourself, add in a few more attempts, up to five per side. Then, you can hold the end position longer every time you do it. Finally, the most challenging version of these is to do these with your arms and legs straight.

But as you've heard before, it's best to focus on the quality of the movement, not just breeze through this exercise as fast as possible. Make each attempt challenging! The goal isn't to progress to the hardest variation.

So working on your core isn't limited to sit-ups! Give this exercise a shot and work on your coordination at the same time.

CORE - BACKSIDE

ONE THING PEOPLE don't consider when doing core work is the importance of the backside. I'm not talking about the muscles in your rear, I'm talking about the entirety of the chain you can't see in the mirror, from the bottom tip of your spine to your shoulder blades.

Core work involves training both front AND back. Our goal is to balance out the quality work we did on the front side of the core using dead bugs with a second move, the cross crawl superman.

The move you're about to see also trains your coordination since it involves lifting opposite limbs at the same time. It's less strenuous move, one that's all about the pattern of the movement, but it still requires you to get down on the floor. This time, lying on your chest/stomach.

SUPERMAN CROSS-CRAWL

An important concept here is reaching. Imagine trying to touch the wall ahead with your fingers and the wall behind with your toes.

Unless you're Mr. Fantastic, it won't
happen, but it's an effective way to
visualize the intent.

It's called the superman because by
lifting up both arms and both legs at
the same time, you look like Christo-
pher Reeves flying through the air!
(Lots of superhero references in this
section.)

This move needs to be performed a
large number of times. Try and
complete ten per side, or twenty
total. More practice means a longer
time to stay focused; try not to get
distracted while you do these. Stay
present while you reach forward and
up with your arms and backward and
up with your legs.

USING YOUR BODY

Remember, your body isn't a
conglomeration of parts. That works for Dr. Frankenstein's monster,
but it's not how you were designed! There are no "abs" of the back, so
there needs to be a more all-encompassing approach.

That's why we use all four of our limbs! A study published in 2013
found that all muscle groups of the backside were more active when
lifting the chest off the floor (the Superman part) when compared to
just lifting the leg. [25] The beauty of this exercise is that we are
doing both!

In addition to recruiting the most possible muscle groups, we are also
working on coordination and learning how to sequence patterns natu-

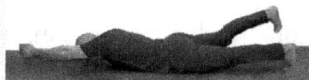

rally built into our system. Ever notice how, when you walk, which-ever leg is forward, the opposite side's arm is lifted?

Like I mentioned before, this exercise isn't as taxing as previous ones. There won't be a time when your muscles are giving out. Movement quality doesn't have to be a struggle!

With this tool in your toolkit, you now have a great one-two punch to approach core work. Don't be surprised when you feel energized after giving these two a shot! It's your body thanking you for the dose of movement.

STANDING TWIST

YOU MIGHT HAVE NOTICED that the core moves we've already learned have been in one line, right down the length of our body.

But what about our sides? You're right, humans don't live on train tracks. Not everything is going to be right down the middle. This section of the core needs to be trained too.

Like we did with the previous exercises focused on the core, we want to incorporate our whole body into the movement. There's going to be a good bit of focus in this move, so make sure you are paying attention while practicing this one!

THE STANDING TWIST

Like the Superman Cross-crawl from the previous section, this move won't be very taxing. But that doesn't mean it's easy! There are a few points you need to focus on.

1. The feet. This one is nuanced, so bear with me. When you twist to the right, maintain contact with the ground with your big toe of the right foot. On the left foot, find the connection of your pinky toe with the ground.

2. When you twist to the left, the big toe on your left foot and the pinky toe on the left foot needs to be in contact with the floor.

3. Your head. Make sure you turn your head as far as you can and *look* at the wall behind you. This means you will be looking out of the side of your eyes.

This attention to detail is why this move is simple but not easy. Pause at a full twist on each side and perform five twists per side.

WHY THE ATTENTION TO DETAIL?

Do you find yourself why any of this matters? You could just twist with reckless abandon, and if you want to, go ahead! Have fun with it, put some music on and have a dance party!

What the above tips do is increase the effectiveness of the movement.

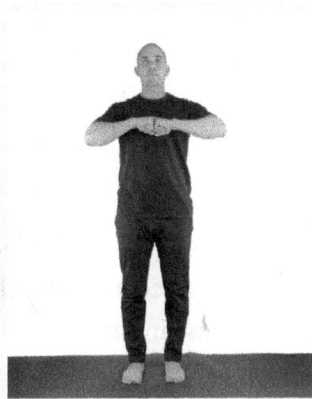

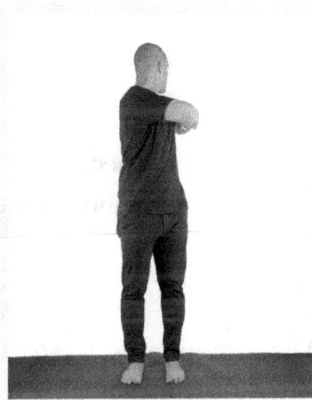

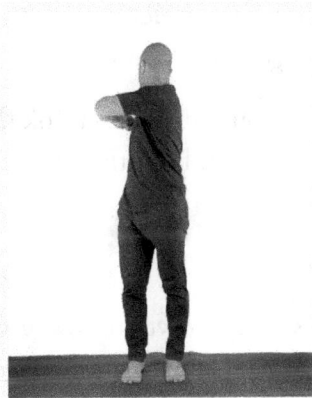

More bang for your buck, if you will. The better the quality, the sooner the results! Plus, the goal of this book is to introduce you to your body and all the beautiful ways it can move. I'd be doing you a disservice if I didn't at least *mention* these tidbits (which I find fascinating by the way).

We want to focus on the feet to strengthen them. A study on a group of 158 adolescents found that excess weight was associated with low muscle mass in the arches of the feet. [26] Another study found that an exercise used to improve the strength of an arch of the foot (there are three arches) also improved the balance of the test subjects. [27,28]

Put simply, strengthening the feet will lead to better balance!

We focus on the head and eyes during this movement because we are trying to get the neck moving. Obesity has been associated with a lack of movement options in the neck, with a recommendation to recruit the neck muscles neck during movement as a preventative measure for pain. [29]

A reduction in neck movement options could also lead to increased activity in the link between your eyes and neck. [30] Increased activity in this link, called the cervical-ocular reflex, has also been shown to be elevated when neck pain is present. [31,32] This is why we get the eyes involved as well!

Bet you didn't ever think there was so much involved with manipulating your body through space, did you?

MIXING IT IN

As with everything we've gone over up to this point, take your time when practicing this movement. Then try to layer it into your daily life with the others we have already reviewed. It's not easy, so start with the ones that speak to you and try those out first. Then, pick your favorites and do them as often as you can. It's ok to cherry-pick when you're just getting started!

Now that we've reviewed both above and below the hips let's move onto exercises moving your whole body in space!

EXERCISE FAMILY 3 - MOVING

GET DOWN

WHEN'S THE last time you got down on the floor?

As a kid, you did it all the time. If you were to walk into a child's classroom or play area, being on the floor is commonplace and expected.

You were on the floor before you started to crawl. Then crawling on the floor before you could walk. But even while learning to walk, you fell, meeting with the ground again.

Take a second to look at the floor now. Does the idea of getting down there seem daunting? Far away?

The goal of this section is to become friends with the floor.

Most adults don't get down on the floor with any sort of regularity, except for playing with children or pets. This means that something as simple as a fall can become catastrophic since your body doesn't have a strategy to get down safely.

Even if you DO find yourself on the floor regularly, this section will show you an exercise that elevates your heart rate and gets you breathing heavily.

GET DOWN... THEN GET BACK UP

The magic happened between the pictures. Use any strategy YOU want, it doesn't matter. I suggest getting down onto your stomach first then rolling onto your back before reversing the process.

If you're standing and unsure of where to start, initiate the movement by getting down onto one knee then putting a hand down. You might want to make sure you're on a carpeted surface or have a yoga mat down, so your knees don't get tender.

There are two ways we can approach this in practice:

1. Get down, then get back up five times. Rest and repeat.
2. Set a timer for one to two minutes and try to stay moving the whole time, getting down as many times as you can. Rest and repeat.

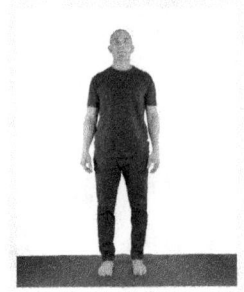

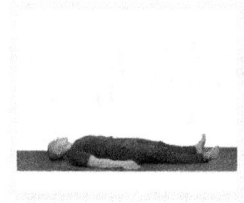

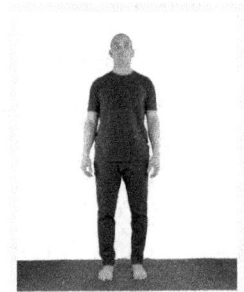

INCREASING THE DIFFICULTY

If this version isn't advanced enough for you, don't worry; there are ways of making it harder.

We'll start by taking an arm out of the equation. Either pin your arm to your chest like this:

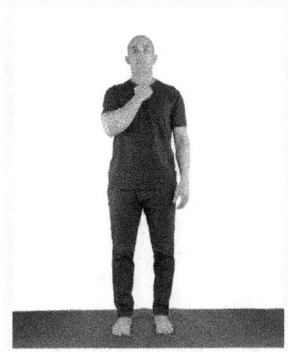

Or hold one arm overhead like this:

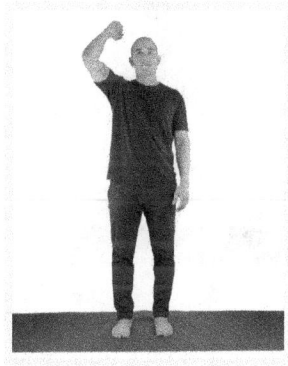

And try to get down onto your back before standing up again. Introduce this variation the same way as before, but be sure to get down and get back up the same number of times on each side.

Another way to increase the difficulty is to "paste" your hand to your knee:

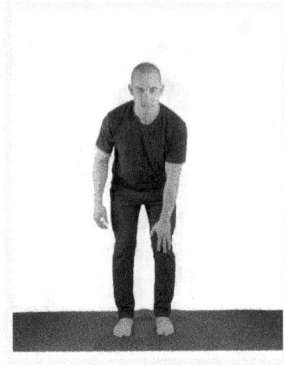

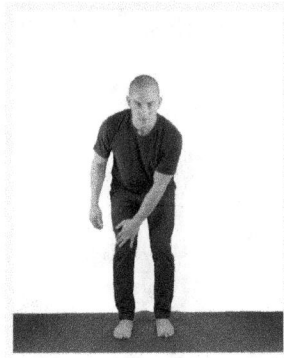

Try and keep your hand in contact with your knee the entire time. This one is demanding, so feel free to let that hand break contact if you need to until you get comfortable.

The most challenging version I'd like to show you is with both hands behind your back:

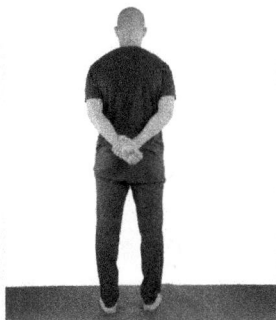

It is possible! It's quite the challenge, but if you feel like you are up to it, then go ahead and give it a shot!

NO EQUIPMENT NECESSARY

This move is great because it can be done *anywhere*. You don't need weights, machines, or even leave the room you're in. This does present its own challenges because it can be difficult to exercise in the same place you relax. If you find yourself struggling to get started, try picking a different area of your home to try this one out.

One way a client found to include this move into their lives: get down and get back up during commercials. It's only a few minutes at a time, but as long as you stay moving the entire time, it will be plenty of time to get quality work in. This also works if you wanted to add this move in between shows.

Sprinkling in this move will get your body ready for more strenuous exercise, get your blood flowing, and will get you comfortable with the ground once more. Over time this will help set the foundation for when you're ready to take on more challenging forms of exercise when bariatric surgery is far in your rearview mirror.

Simple yet effective!

BABY CRAWL

WHAT IF I told you that your newfound comfort with the floor has unlocked a way to exercise every body part? Not just your legs, shoulders, and core, but your coordination as well.

The best part, still no machines or weights required!

Up to now, we haven't introduced any external load to the movements we have practiced. The shoulders, in particular, could stand with a little more work, don't you think? And no, we aren't going to do push-ups or planks.

Our goal is to work on shoulder strength and stability by adding weight while moving. To do so, we're taking it old school, back to when you were a young one.

BABY CRAWL

The best way to think about this movement is to move opposite limbs at the same time. Take a quick pause at each position to keep your arms and legs in sync. Pretend some-one's taking a picture of you each time!

We keep the arm straight while we do these so that the shoulders are doing the work to stabilize our bodies. Once you take one hand off the floor, you are increasing the amount of weight being supported by the arm still on the floor in a way that is safe and effective. Your other arm is always there in case you need addi-tional support.

Notice how my eyes are ahead of me, looking out at the horizon. Keep your eyes on a spot ahead at the same height as your head. Resist the urge to look down at your body! Your limbs don't need you to witness them moving to move correctly. I promise you, you'll be the first to know if some-thing happens to your arms or legs.

To add this move in, set a timer for anywhere from one to five minutes then try to stay moving the whole time. Rest and repeat.

COMMON ISSUES

There are two significant issues people have when introducing crawling for the first time:

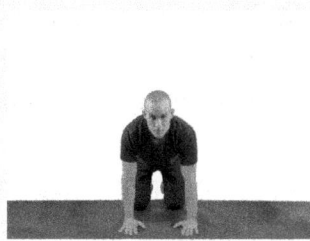

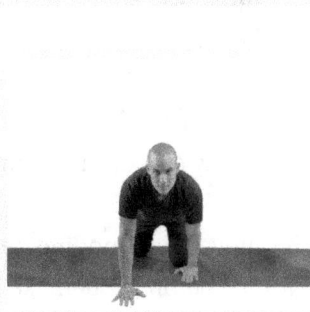

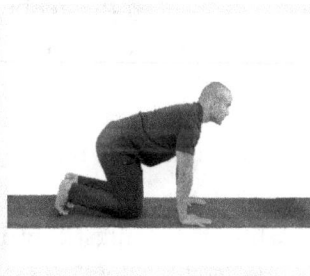

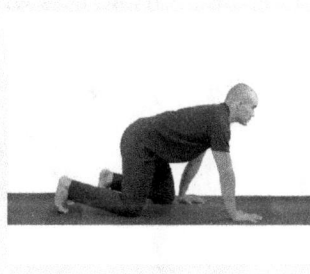

1. Knee pain. This happens because of the pressure on the knees from being on the ground. Use a carpeted area. If crawling is still painful, call it quits for the day. Try again when the knee pain subsides.
2. Limb sequencing. Most of the time, this happens because the steps are being taken too quickly. Slow down, and don't forget the pause at each position. This can also occur because the steps with the legs/knees are too big, forcing the hand that should be planted to come off the ground early. Lots of small steps are better than taking giant steps that throw off your rhythm

This move might not feel terribly taxing when you perform it but give it a day before you make your conclusions. The residual soreness usually shows up in the shoulders as a feeling like your back or neck needs to crack. If this feeling does show up, make sure it's gone before you try crawling again. It shouldn't take more than a few days to disappear.

Crawling is a move that will stick with you for the long haul. Even if you get to the point of training push-ups and exercises with weights, crawling is a fantastic warm-up. It helps keep your shoulder joint healthy, stable, and able to move. Plus, getting down and playing with young children and pets will be no problem at all!

WALKING

ONE OF THE problems with the exercises we've discussed so far is scalability. Everything we've encountered up to now can be measured by both time and number of repetitions performed. By practicing consistently, the amount of work done within a given time can improve.

But, without weights, there is a point where you get good enough at these exercises; they become more qualitative in nature.

For example, once you stand up and sit down well enough, how do you continue to improve?

Or, if you can crawl for five minutes at a time at a consistent speed, there isn't much more you can do other than focus on getting better at the movement itself.

Simply put, once you learn these exercises, there are diminishing returns on performing them longer and for more repetitions.

The goal of this book is to provide exercises you can perform at home. Without introducing weights. Therefore, I want to add an activity that you can scale up for both increased time intervals and higher repetition counts.

WALKING

Walking has seen a resurgence with the rise of wearable fitness trackers. There are all sorts of recommendations about how many steps should be performed each day.

My recommendation: more. It doesn't matter where you start, just get your body moving. If you've done the exercises up to this point, your joints and tissues are set up for success.

To be clear, I'm not suggesting you get a wearable fitness tracker. My goal in mentioning the technology was to address the fact that there are numerous sources about how much is the "correct" amount.

Walking is great because it provides straightforward markers for improvement. Did you walk for a longer time interval? Did you go further (a measure of your number of steps)?

Just like the rest of the exercises we perform, it's not about how much you can get done at once, or in a day; it's about how many days in a row you can show up and put in the work. *Consistency* is the name of the game.

Don't have any value assigned to how far or how long you go. Just get some steps in and be ready to come back next time.

THE PLAN

To start regularly walking, you don't even need to leave your house. Don't believe me? I've heard many stories of people trying to get their steps in for the day while watching tv! One client paces the length of their living room until they get the step count according to their wearable.

My suggestion is for you to start in the same place. Literally. Remember the paused marching exercise from Exercise Family 1? We're going to do the same thing without the focus on knee height. You can watch tv, talk on the phone, or listen to music/podcast/audiobook. But stay standing and keep those feet moving!

When you're tired, rest. If you feel up to it, try for another round. Whenever you want to call it a day, go ahead... but keep in mind your goal to try again next time.

Once you've outgrown marching in place, begin pacing the room. Or walking between rooms. You might not be able to watch tv anymore, but you can still talk on the phone or listen to audio!

Both marching in place and taking steps in the house are based on how long you perform the task. There's no reason to monitor your step count.

Finally, take it outside and go for a walk when you're ready! It can be tempting to go out for a walk and turn around when you feel tired but keep in mind, you'll still need to come back! It's better to pick a set distance and do laps, maybe on your driveway or street, until you get a solid grasp on how long you can walk before you've had enough.

CONSISTENCY

I've said this a few times already but wanted to bring it up once more. Don't worry about the results. How long and how far you walk doesn't matter; it's about sticking to the schedule and maintaining a movement habit.

Three times a week is an excellent place to start. Give your body time to recover and notice any soreness. This will go away once your body becomes used to consistent work output. One day you'll realize it's gone. That's how you'll know when it's time to push for more time or distance.

At first, the proof you're getting better shows up in how easy the task becomes to perform. It's a qualitative measurement. Once you go for longer or further, it becomes a quantitive measurement.

Please ignore the urge to search for improvement until you've established the habit. It will pay off in the long run.

Focusing on consistency will snowball to the rest of your movement practice. You might be wondering how to implement all that you've learned so far. That's the final section!

You now have all the tools in your toolkit. Let's move on to designing what a complete workout might look like.

PUTTING IT ALL TOGETHER

MAKING YOUR WORKOUT

AT THIS POINT, we've covered A LOT of ground. Your head might be swirling, wondering how on Earth you're supposed to do all of these exercises every day.

The short answer: you're not.

If you are feeling overwhelmed by the prospect of doing all these exercises every day, please keep reading! I'm going to provide you with an actionable plan in three easy to implement templates.

By the end of this, you'll have a much better sense of how long each workout should take, and how often they should be completed, and what the structure looks like.

KEEP FIGHTING

I'll say it up front: there's too much content in this book to be performed in one workout. So we aren't even going to try.

While it may seem like I'm cutting you some slack, please keep in mind that even top athletes rotate the exercises they perform within a given span of days or weeks. Splitting up the week is normal!

Instead of fitting everything into one workout, I want you to split the exercises from the three families up into three separate days. Each is designed to take half an hour.

These templates are all time-based. Don't worry about how many times each exercise is completed in the intervals below, just do your best to stay moving the entire time.

Workout Template 1

Spend 2:00 on 2 exercises from {Exercise Family 1} and 2 from {Exercise Family 2}. Rest 1:00 between each 2:00 interval and repeat.

The above section takes 23:00. You'll rest 2:00 then perform 5:00 practicing 1 exercise from {Exercise Family 3}.

Pick any ones you like for day one, it doesn't matter. For Example:

A.

2:00 Single Leg Balancing

1:00 Rest

2:00 Paused Marching

1:00 Rest

2:00 Core - Frontside

1:00 Rest

2:00 Standing Twist

1:00 Rest

Repeat, then Rest 2:00

B.

5:00 Baby Crawl

Workout Template 2

Pick one exercise from each family. Then you'll work for 1:00 and rest for a 1:00 interval, cycling through the movements.

Example:

1:00 Stand Up, Sit Down

1:00 Rest

1:00 Shoulders (any variation)

1:00 Rest

1:00 Get Down

1:00 Rest

Repeat 5 times.

Note: This template also works without cycling through the different exercises. For example, all five work intervals (with rest between) of Stand Up, Sit Down before moving onto the Shoulders (any variation)

Workout Template 3

Pick one exercise from each family. Then you'll work for 10:00 on one at a time, any way you like while working at your own pace and resting as needed.

Example:

10:00 Bending at the hip

10:00 Core - Backside

10:00 Walking

Workout Template 4

Spend 6:00 on 4 exercises from the twelve available in {Exercise Family 1-3}. Rest 2:00 between each 6:00 interval. Pick at least one exercise from each family.

Example:

6:00 Standing Knee Bends

2:00 Rest

6:00 Bending at the hip

2:00 Rest

6:00 Shoulders (any variation)

2:00 Rest

6:00 Get Down

PUTTING TOGETHER YOUR WEEK

The goal is to try and perform a half-hour workout three times a week. Use whichever workout templates you prefer, and the same one multiple times if you want. Just make sure you perform all twelve exercises within a given week.

Be careful, some of the templates only use three of the exercises and performing workouts with just these templates won't get all twelve completed.

It's ok to repeat exercises throughout the week, so if you like one, add it in multiple times!

If life gets in the way, it might be tempting to quit... why bother if the goal can't be achieved? Well, something is better than nothing. Do what you can! If it turns out to be twice a week, or if your workouts get cut short, just be ready to come back and try again next time.

Do yourself a favor and stick to the plan. Perform what you set out to do before you decide if it's too much or not enough. You might surprise yourself with your ability to show up next time, or alternatively, you might find out that you aren't recovering as well as you'd hoped.

This becomes especially important when adding an extra workout within the week. Don't decide mid-week to add the day. Stick to the original plan, complete the week, then develop a new strategy for the following week.

These four templates are your starting point to bring all the movements together. In time you might be able to start adding in more walking, but when it comes to the exercises themselves, think long term. Little chunks of practice over a long time add up!

You are ready to get started. You can do this, one half-hour chunk at a time.

KEEPING THE HABIT

BUILDING AND KEEPING POSITIVE HABITS, like exercise, doesn't happen overnight. It takes time, patience, and a fair amount of self-forgiveness until new habits become second nature.

The initial battle against inertia is some of the hardest steps to take.

No matter how much you *want* to show up each and every day, old patterns are hard to break. They're comfortable. Familiar. What's the point of a comfort zone if not to stay warm and cozy inside?

At a certain point, motivation will give out. It's a fact. Nobody who exercises with regularity is chomping at the bit each and every day. This is where dedication comes into play.

Motivation is the desire to start a task. If you're reading this, I'm going to assume you want to get started and are looking for guidance.

Dedication is a commitment to engage in the desired behaviors.

It seems like a small difference, but it's an important one. Motivation is fleeting. It goes away as soon as the obstacles loom too large. Motivation is internal. On the other hand, dedication is a commitment to the actions, an addition to the inner desire.

THE BEST WAY TO BUILD THE HABIT

I'd like to discuss some methods my clients have found to be useful to incorporate exercise into their daily routines.

The first step is to decide the goal. To start, shoot for three days a week of dedicated practice to the movements mentioned in this book. Make a plan *before* the week begins regarding which days are going to be the ones you exercise. I suggest Monday, Wednesday, Friday to start. If your job leaves you little time at home, pick one day during the week, Wednesday, for example, and then plan to move on both Saturday and Sunday.

Stick to the plan without judgment. It's much more vital *that* you move, not how you move.

Cross off days

This simple method is the one my clients have found works best. Get a calendar and cross off the days you complete your movement practice. Ideally, these align with the plan you set out for the week, but it's ok if the workout falls on other days. The important thing is to get three days crossed off in a week. Then, come back the next week and repeat the effort.

Build up while motivation is high and carry on with the habit when dedication is required.

One client found that crossing off the day the night before the planned movement day worked best for them. This made sure they got the work done because they had already crossed off the day.

Whichever way you choose to incorporate this strategy, the point is to accumulate enough crossed off days until you have momentum that can't be broken. This one is also especially good for daily tasks, like drinking a glass of water in the morning, so the string of continuous crossed off days is more recognizable.

One pitfall of this method is when a day or week isn't crossed off the way you planned. When this happens, give yourself a break and make a promise to try again next time. It's ok the fail, it's not ok to not learn the lesson failure has to offer.

Get an accountability partner

This method works great if there is someone in your life that you trust to keep up with your progress judgment-free. Inform them each time you finish a workout to let them know you showed up and did the work.

It might be hard to let someone know you're on this journey, but I promise you they'll be rooting for you!

One pitfall from this method is that you may come to feel resentment towards the other person. Don't let their expectations weigh you down! Avoidance is the worst-case scenario. Still talk to them, explain what happened and how you'll fix the situation next time. If they aren't supportive, then consider finding a new accountability partner.

Use an app

Similar to an accountability partner, this method relies on technology to help make sure you show up each day.

If you don't mind sharing, there are thousands of people in the world who would love to encourage you on your journey. Find a Facebook group of people in similar circumstances and check in regularly.

Or, create your own content on social media. Facebook posts and Instagram videos that share your progress can inspire others to follow in your footsteps.

If sharing isn't your thing, use your phone's camera to make a video for yourself. Looking back on the progress you make is a great way to realize how your hard work is paying off!

GETTING INTO THE RHYTHM

Motivation makes the first day, or first week, the easiest. It isn't hard to move when you're chomping at the bit and fired up to get started.

The second... well, that's a different story. The real battle begins when the initial desire cools. Can you still show up, do the work, when you don't feel like it?

Start small, with a manageable plan, keeping in mind that all movement is a successful day. Starting small will allow you to get the snowball rolling, and over time it becomes an unstoppable force.

It comes down to a decision that you make once it isn't easy or fun anymore. Will you keep showing up?

Just like the moves in this book, practicing moving when you don't feel like it will get easier as you get better at the skill. Your capacity will increase, causing small roadblocks of low motivation to seem trivial in the future. Your willingness to move will be affected less and less by situations that might have derailed you before.

You just have to start.

Once you do, you can use these methods to cultivate other positive habits. Drinking water and reading are my suggestions, but ask yourself, what would **you** like to add to your own routine?

You just have to start.

ONE STEP AT A TIME

WE'VE MADE it to the end of the book.

My hope is that you found this informative, actionable, and manageable.

If you're still not sure where to start, pick one of the moves that interested you and give it a shot! See how well you do. Set a baseline and find out how much better you can get with a little practice.

Then follow the steps in here to create your very own movement practice. One that will help you regardless of if you're preparing for bariatric surgery or if you've already undergone the procedure.

Moving may seem daunting, and there's a chance you want to wait until the weight is gone to get started. Remember my words from earlier in this book: you can learn how to move regardless of your physical size. Don't let the images of people you see as "typical" exercisers affect your opinion of your abilities. Humans are designed with the same basic structure, so age and physical size don't change whether you can perform the moves in this book.

You can take control of your ability to move. These are the steps. Take one at a time, and you'll be on your way!

REFERENCES

1. Respiratory Management of Perioperative Obese Patients
2. Respiratory Pattern of Diaphragmatic Breathing and Pilates Breathing in COPD Subjects
3. Diaphragm and lungs
4. Diaphragmatic Amplitude and Accessory Inspiratory Muscle Activity in Nasal and Mouth-Breathing Adults: A Cross-Sectional Study
5. Tongue Pressure Measurement in Children With Mouth-Breathing Behaviour
6. Tongue Protrusion Strength in Arousal State Is Predictive of the Airway Patency in Obstructive Sleep Apnea
7. Weight Loss and Obesity in the Treatment and Prevention of Osteoarthritis
8. Obesity indices and inflammatory markers in obese non-diabetic normo- and hypertensive patients: a comparative pilot study
9. The evolving role of obesity in knee osteoarthritis
10. Increased Daily Movement Associates With Reduced

Mortality Among COPD Patients Having Systemic
Inflammation

11. Effects of Obesity on Balance and Gait Alterations in
Young Adults

12. The Effects of Toe-Out and Toe-In Postures on Static &
Dynamic Balance, Risk of Fall and TUG Score in Healthy
Adults

13. The impact of obesity on balance control in community-
dwelling older women

14. Obesity, Muscular Strength, Muscle Composition and
Physical Performance in an Elderly Population

15. Effects of a walking exercise program for obese individuals
with intellectual disability staying in a residential care
facility

16. Three-dimensional Gait Analysis of Obese Adults

17. Prevalence of Self-Reported Pain, Joint Complaints and
Knee or Hip Complaints in Adults Aged ≥ 40 Years: A
Cross-Sectional Survey in Herne, Germany

18. Six degree-of-freedom knee joint kinematics in obese
individuals with knee pain during gait

19. The Association Between Obesity and Low Back Pain and
Disability Is Affected by Mood Disorders

20. The role of obesity in the biomechanics and radiological
changes of the spine: an in vitro study

21. The Epidemiology of Low Back Pain

22. Strength Training: Isometric Training at a Range of Joint
Angles Versus Dynamic Training

23. Obesity Effect on Male Active Joint Range of Motion

24. Lumbar Spine Stability Can Be Augmented With an
Abdominal Belt and/or Increased Intra-Abdominal Pressure

25. Posterior muscle chain activity during various extension
exercises: an observational study

26. Body Fat and Muscle Mass in Association with Foot
Structure in Adolescents: A Cross-Sectional Study

27. The effects of short foot exercises and arch support insoles on improvement in the medial longitudinal arch and dynamic balance of flexible flatfoot patients

28. Immediate Effect of Short-foot Exercise on Dynamic Balance of Subjects With Excessively Pronated Feet

29. Impact of Fat Infiltration in Cervical Extensor Muscles on Cervical Lordosis and Neck Pain: A Cross-Sectional Study

30. The Influence of Cervical Movement on Eye Stabilization Reflexes: A Randomized Trial

31. Eye Stabilization Reflexes in Traumatic and Non-Traumatic Chronic Neck Pain Patients

32. Cervico-ocular Reflex Is Increased in People With Nonspecific Neck Pain

ABOUT THE AUTHOR

Marcos Hernandez is an author and movement coach based in the suburbs of Washington, D.C.

Marcos graduated from the University of Maryland, College Park with a degree in chemical engineering and a minor in physics. Since graduating, he has worked as a barista, a food scientist, and a CrossFit coach.

www.ingramcontent.com/pod-product-compliance
Lightning Source LLC
Chambersburg PA
CBHW050543280326
41933CB00011B/1694